THE GRASS FED DIET COOKBOOK

NATAELIE BROWN

Copyright ©2024.

All rights reserved. No part of this publication may be reproduced, distributed, or transmitted in any form or by any means, including photocopying, recording, or other electronic or mechanical methods, without the prior written permission of the publisher, except in the case of brief quotations embodied in critical reviews and certain other non commercial uses permitted by copyright law

TABLE OF CONTENTS

WHAT IS GRAVE DISEASE 3

IMPORTANCE OF NUTRITION 4

FOODS TO EAT 5

FOODS TO AVOID 7

14 DAYS MEAL PLAN FOR GRAVES DISEASE 9

BREAKFAST RECIPES FOR GRAVES' DISEASE COOKBOOK 16

LUNCH RECIPES FOR GRAVES' DISEASE COOKBOOK 22

DINNER RECIPES FOR GRAVES' DISEASE COOKBOOK 29

SNACK AND SWEET RECIPES FOR GRAVES' DISEASE COOKBOOK 38

BEVERAGE AND SMOOTHIE RECIPES FOR GRAVES' DISEASE COOKBOOK 43

CONCLUSION 49

WHAT IS GRAVE DISEASE

Graves' disease manifests in a myriad of ways, disrupting the delicate balance of the body's hormone production. Its symptoms are diverse, ranging from the physical—such as weight loss or gain, palpitations, tremors, and heat intolerance—to the emotional—like anxiety, mood swings, and fatigue. This complex interplay can significantly impact daily life, requiring a comprehensive approach to management. Graves' disease, a thyroid disorder characterized by an overactive thyroid gland, introduces unique challenges. From fluctuations in metabolism to potential impacts on overall health, the complexities demand a holistic approach. As such, this cookbook aims not only to offer delicious recipes but also to serve as a guide, empowering individuals to make informed dietary choices.

IMPORTANCE OF NUTRITION

Nutrition stands as a cornerstone in the multifaceted management of Graves' disease. The food we consume has a profound impact, not only on our overall health but specifically on the functioning of the thyroid gland. The right dietary choices can complement medical interventions, alleviate symptoms, and promote a sense of well-being.

FOODS TO EAT

1. **Nutrient-Dense Vegetables**

   - Leafy Greens: Spinach, kale, Swiss chard, and broccoli offer essential vitamins and minerals like folate and vitamin K.
   - Colorful Veggies: Carrots, bell peppers, and sweet potatoes provide antioxidants like beta-carotene and vitamin C.

2. **Lean Proteins**

   - Poultry: Chicken and turkey offer high-quality protein and are leaner options compared to red meat.
   - Fish: Salmon, mackerel, and sardines are rich in omega-3 fatty acids, beneficial for heart health and inflammation.

3. **Whole Grains**

   - Quinoa, Brown Rice, and Oats: These whole grains provide fiber, essential for digestive health, and have a lower impact on blood sugar levels.

4. Healthy Fats

- Avocado: Rich in monounsaturated fats, vitamins, and minerals, it supports heart health and provides essential nutrients.
- Nuts and Seeds: Almonds, walnuts, chia seeds, and flaxseeds offer omega-3 fatty acids and are excellent sources of protein.

5. Dairy Alternatives

- Almond Milk, Coconut Yogurt: For those sensitive to dairy, these alternatives offer calcium and are lower in lactose.

6. Antioxidant-Rich Fruits

- Berries: Blueberries, strawberries, and raspberries provide antioxidants that combat inflammation and support overall health.
- Citrus Fruits: Oranges, lemons, and grapefruits offer vitamin C, supporting the immune system.

FOODS TO AVOID

1. Iodine-Rich Foods

Seafood: High iodine content in seaweed, shrimp, and iodized salt may exacerbate symptoms of hyperthyroidism.

2. Caffeine and Stimulants

Coffee, Tea, and Energy Drinks: Stimulants can worsen symptoms like palpitations and anxiety associated with Graves' disease.

3. Processed and Refined Foods

Fast Food, Sugary Treats: These foods are often high in unhealthy fats, sugar, and preservatives, contributing to inflammation.

4. Soy-Based Products

Soybeans, Tofu: These contain compounds that may interfere with thyroid function; moderation is recommended.

5. Excessive Sugar and Artificial Sweeteners

Sodas, Candies: High sugar intake can lead to energy fluctuations and weight gain, affecting overall health.

Artificial Sweeteners: Some may impact thyroid function; opting for natural alternatives like stevia can be a better choice.

6. Gluten

Wheat-Based Products: Some individuals with autoimmune conditions may benefit from reducing gluten intake, though evidence is mixed.

14 DAYS MEAL PLAN FOR GRAVES DISEASE

Day 1

- Breakfast: Greek yogurt with mixed berries and a sprinkle of chia seeds
- Snack: Apple slices with almond butter
- Lunch: Quinoa salad with spinach, cherry tomatoes, cucumbers, and grilled chicken
- Snack: Carrot sticks with hummus
- Dinner: Baked salmon with roasted sweet potatoes and steamed broccoli

Day 2

- Breakfast: Spinach and mushroom omelette with whole-grain toast
- Snack: Handful of mixed nuts
- Lunch: Lentil soup with a side of mixed green salad
- Snack: Greek yogurt with honey and walnuts
- Dinner: Turkey meatballs with zucchini noodles and marinara sauce

Day 3

- Breakfast: Green smoothie (kale, banana, almond milk, and protein powder)
- Snack: Sliced cucumber with cottage cheese
- Lunch: Grilled shrimp salad with mixed greens, avocado, and citrus vinaigrette
- Snack: Rice cakes with avocado spread
- Dinner: Stir-fried tofu with bell peppers, snap peas, and brown rice

Day 4

- Breakfast: Overnight oats with almond milk, topped with sliced almonds and diced apples
- Snack: Celery sticks with peanut butter
- Lunch: Quinoa-stuffed bell peppers with a side of mixed greens
- Snack: Berries with a dollop of Greek yogurt
- Dinner: Grilled chicken breast with roasted Brussels sprouts and quinoa

Day 5

- Breakfast: Greek yogurt parfait with granola and mixed berries
- Snack: Trail mix (nuts and dried fruits)
- Lunch: Chickpea salad with cucumber, cherry tomatoes, feta cheese, and lemon-tahini dressing
- Snack: Cottage cheese with pineapple chunks
- Dinner: Baked cod with steamed asparagus and wild rice

Day 6

- Breakfast: Whole-grain toast with avocado and poached eggs
- Snack: Apple slices with cinnamon
- Lunch: Turkey and vegetable stir-fry with brown rice
- Snack: Rice cakes with almond butter
- Dinner: Lentil curry with spinach and a side of quinoa

Day 7

- Breakfast: Spinach and feta crustless quiche
- Snack: Handful of pumpkin seeds
- Lunch: Mixed bean salad with bell peppers, red onion, and a balsamic vinaigrette
- Snack: Carrot sticks with hummus
- Dinner: Grilled sirloin steak with roasted sweet potato wedges and steamed green beans

Day 8

- Breakfast: Berry and spinach smoothie bowl topped with nuts and seeds
- Snack: Sliced cucumber with cottage cheese
- Lunch: Tuna salad lettuce wraps with diced veggies
- Snack: Berries with a dollop of Greek yogurt
- Dinner: Chicken and vegetable kebabs with a side of quinoa salad

Day 9

- Breakfast: Chia seed pudding with coconut milk and sliced mango
- Snack: Handful of mixed nuts
- Lunch: Roasted vegetable and quinoa bowl with tahini dressing
- Snack: Rice cakes with avocado spread
- Dinner: Baked tofu with sautéed bok choy and brown rice

Day 10

- Breakfast: Overnight oats with almond milk, topped with sliced almonds and diced peaches
- Snack: Celery sticks with hummus
- Lunch: Spinach and feta stuffed chicken breast with a side of roasted vegetables
- Snack: Apple slices with almond butter
- Dinner: Grilled shrimp skewers with quinoa and a green salad

Day 11

- Breakfast: Greek yogurt with mixed berries and a sprinkle of granola
- Snack: Handful of pumpkin seeds
- Lunch: Black bean and sweet potato chili
- Snack: Carrot sticks with hummus
- Dinner: Lemon herb roasted chicken with steamed broccoli and wild rice

Day 12

- Breakfast: Spinach and mushroom frittata
- Snack: Mixed nuts and dried fruit
- Lunch: Zucchini noodles with marinara sauce and turkey meatballs
- Snack: Rice cakes with almond butter
- Dinner: Baked cod with quinoa and sautéed spinach

Day 13

- Breakfast: Avocado toast with poached eggs and cherry tomatoes
- Snack: Greek yogurt with honey and walnuts
- Lunch: Lentil and vegetable stir-fry with brown rice

- Snack: Berries with a dollop of Greek yogurt
- Dinner: Grilled steak salad with mixed greens and balsamic vinaigrette

Day 14

- Breakfast: Whole-grain pancakes with fresh fruit and a drizzle of honey
- Snack: Sliced cucumber with cottage cheese
- Lunch: Quinoa-stuffed bell peppers with a side of mixed greens
- Snack: Trail mix (nuts and dried fruits)
- Dinner: Baked salmon with roasted asparagus and quinoa

BREAKFAST RECIPES FOR GRAVES' DISEASE COOKBOOK

AVOCADO TOAST WITH POACHED EGGS

INGREDIENTS:

- Whole-grain bread
- Ripe avocado
- Eggs
- Salt and pepper to taste

INSTRUCTIONS:

1. Toast the whole-grain bread to your desired level of crispness.
2. Mash the ripe avocado and spread it evenly on the toast.
3. Prepare poached eggs and place them on top of the avocado.
4. Season with salt and pepper. Enjoy!

BERRY AND SPINACH SMOOTHIE BOWL

INGREDIENTS:

- Spinach
- Mixed berries (fresh or frozen)
- Almond milk (or any preferred milk)
- Greek yogurt (optional)
- Nuts, seeds, or granola for topping

INSTRUCTIONS:

1. Blend spinach, mixed berries, almond milk, and Greek yogurt until smooth.
2. Pour the smoothie into a bowl.
3. Top with nuts, seeds, or granola for added texture and flavor.

CHIA SEED PUDDING

INGREDIENTS:

- Chia seeds
- Coconut milk (or any preferred milk)
- Honey or maple syrup
- Sliced mango or berries for topping

INSTRUCTIONS:

1. Mix chia seeds with coconut milk and sweeten with honey or maple syrup.
2. Stir well and let it sit in the refrigerator overnight.
3. Top with sliced mango or berries before serving.

GREEK YOGURT PARFAIT

INGREDIENTS:

- Greek yogurt
- Mixed berries
- Chia seeds
- Honey or agave (optional)

INSTRUCTIONS:

1. Layer Greek yogurt with mixed berries and sprinkle chia seeds in between.
2. Drizzle with honey or agave for added sweetness if desired.

GREEN SMOOTHIE BOWL

INGREDIENTS:

- Spinach
- Banana
- Almond milk
- Protein powder (optional)
- Nuts, seeds, or fresh fruit for topping

INSTRUCTIONS:

1. Blend spinach, banana, almond milk, and protein powder until smooth.
2. Pour into a bowl and top with nuts, seeds, or fresh fruit.

GREEK YOGURT WITH MIXED BERRIES

INGREDIENTS:

- Greek yogurt
- Mixed berries
- Nuts or seeds for topping

INSTRUCTIONS:

1. Spoon Greek yogurt into a bowl.
2. Top with mixed berries and sprinkle nuts or seeds on top for added crunch.

OVERNIGHT OATS

INGREDIENTS:

- Rolled oats
- Almond milk
- Chia seeds
- Diced fruits (e.g., apples, peaches)

INSTRUCTIONS:

1. Mix rolled oats, almond milk, chia seeds, and diced fruits in a jar.
2. Refrigerate overnight. Enjoy it cold in the morning.

SPINACH AND FETA CRUSTLESS QUICHE

INGREDIENTS:

- Eggs
- Spinach
- Feta cheese
- Diced tomatoes

INSTRUCTIONS:

1. Preheat oven. Whisk eggs and combine with spinach, feta cheese, and diced tomatoes.
2. Pour into a baking dish and bake until set. Serve warm.

SPINACH AND MUSHROOM OMELETTE

INGREDIENTS:

- Eggs
- Spinach
- Mushrooms
- Feta cheese (optional)

INSTRUCTIONS:

1. Beat eggs in a bowl. Sauté spinach and mushrooms in a pan.
2. Pour beaten eggs into the pan and cook until set. Add feta cheese if desired.

WHOLE-GRAIN PANCAKES

INGREDIENTS:

- Whole-grain flour
- Fresh fruit (e.g., berries, bananas)
- Honey or pure maple syrup

INSTRUCTIONS:

1. Prepare pancake batter using whole-grain flour.
2. Cook pancakes on a griddle. Serve with fresh fruit and a drizzle of honey or maple syrup.

LUNCH RECIPES FOR GRAVES' DISEASE COOKBOOK

CHICKPEA AND SPINACH SALAD

INGREDIENTS:

- Chickpeas
- Spinach
- Cherry tomatoes
- Cucumber
- Feta cheese (optional)
- Lemon-tahini dressing

INSTRUCTIONS:

1. Combine chickpeas, spinach, cherry tomatoes, and sliced cucumber in a bowl.
2. Add crumbled feta cheese if desired.
3. Drizzle with lemon-tahini dressing before serving.

QUINOA STUFFED BELL PEPPERS

INGREDIENTS:

- Quinoa
- Bell peppers
- Mixed vegetables (e.g., corn, peas, carrots)
- Tomato sauce or marinara
- Cheese (optional)

INSTRUCTIONS:

1. Cook quinoa according to package instructions.
2. Mix cooked quinoa with mixed vegetables and tomato sauce.
3. Stuff the mixture into halved bell peppers, sprinkle with cheese if desired, and bake until peppers are tender.

MEDITERRANEAN TUNA SALAD WRAPS

INGREDIENTS:

- Canned tuna
- Cucumbers
- Cherry tomatoes
- Red onion
- Kalamata olives
- Whole-grain wraps

INSTRUCTIONS:

1. Mix canned tuna with diced cucumbers, cherry tomatoes, red onion, and sliced Kalamata olives.
2. Spoon the mixture onto whole-grain wraps and roll them up to make wraps.

GRILLED CHICKEN AND VEGETABLE QUINOA BOWL

INGREDIENTS:

- Grilled chicken breast
- Mixed vegetables (bell peppers, zucchini, etc.)
- Cooked quinoa
- Olive oil
- Lemon juice

INSTRUCTIONS:

1. Grill chicken breast and chop it into pieces.
2. Sauté mixed vegetables in olive oil.
3. Assemble cooked quinoa, grilled chicken, and sautéed vegetables in a bowl. Drizzle with lemon juice.

LENTIL AND VEGETABLE STIR-FRY

INGREDIENTS:

- Cooked lentils
- Assorted vegetables (broccoli, bell peppers, carrots)
- Soy sauce or tamari
- Garlic and ginger (minced)
- Sesame oil

INSTRUCTIONS:

1. Stir-fry assorted vegetables in sesame oil until slightly tender.
2. Add cooked lentils, minced garlic, and ginger.
3. Season with soy sauce or tamari. Stir until combined and heated through.

GREEK QUINOA SALAD

INGREDIENTS:

- Quinoa
- Cucumber
- Cherry tomatoes
- Red onion
- Kalamata olives
- Feta cheese

- Lemon vinaigrette

INSTRUCTIONS:

1. Cook quinoa according to package instructions.
2. Mix cooked quinoa with diced cucumber, cherry tomatoes, sliced red onion, Kalamata olives, and crumbled feta cheese.
3. Drizzle with lemon vinaigrette before serving.

TURKEY AND VEGETABLE STIR-FRY

INGREDIENTS:

- Sliced turkey breast
- Bell peppers
- Snap peas
- Onion
- Soy sauce or tamari
- Rice or quinoa

INSTRUCTIONS:

1. Stir-fry sliced turkey breast with assorted vegetables in a pan.
2. Add soy sauce or tamari for seasoning.
3. Serve over cooked rice or quinoa.

SALMON AND AVOCADO SALAD

INGREDIENTS:

- Grilled or baked salmon fillet
- Mixed greens
- Avocado
- Cherry tomatoes
- Lemon-tahini dressing

INSTRUCTIONS:

1. Place grilled or baked salmon on a bed of mixed greens.
2. Add sliced avocado and cherry tomatoes.
3. Drizzle with lemon-tahini dressing before serving.

MUSHROOM AND SPINACH QUESADILLAS

INGREDIENTS:

- Whole-grain tortillas
- Mushrooms
- Spinach
- Shredded cheese
- Olive oil

INSTRUCTIONS:

1. Sauté mushrooms and spinach in olive oil until wilted.
2. Spread the mixture on one side of a tortilla, sprinkle with shredded cheese, and fold in half.
3. Cook the quesadilla on a skillet until both sides are golden and the cheese is melted.

LENTIL TOMATO SOUP

INGREDIENTS:

- Lentils
- Diced tomatoes
- Carrots
- Celery
- Vegetable broth
- Herbs and spices (such as thyme, garlic powder, paprika)

INSTRUCTIONS:

1. Cook lentils in vegetable broth until tender.
2. Sauté diced tomatoes, carrots, and celery in a pot.

3. Add cooked lentils, vegetable broth, herbs, and spices. Simmer until vegetables are soft and flavors meld.

DINNER RECIPES FOR GRAVES' DISEASE COOKBOOK

BAKED SALMON WITH ROASTED VEGETABLES

INGREDIENTS:

- Salmon fillets
- Assorted vegetables (such as broccoli, bell peppers, and carrots)
- Olive oil
- Lemon juice
- Herbs and spices (e.g., garlic powder, paprika)

INSTRUCTIONS:

1. Season salmon fillets with olive oil, lemon juice, herbs, and spices.
2. Place seasoned salmon on a baking sheet.

3. Toss assorted vegetables in olive oil, season with herbs and spices, and spread them on the same baking sheet.
4. Bake in the oven until the salmon is cooked through and the vegetables are tender.

GRILLED CHICKEN WITH QUINOA AND STEAMED GREENS

INGREDIENTS:

- Chicken breast
- Quinoa
- Assorted greens (spinach, kale, or Swiss chard)
- Olive oil
- Lemon
- Herbs for seasoning

INSTRUCTIONS:

1. Marinate chicken breast with olive oil, lemon juice, and herbs.
2. Grill the chicken until fully cooked.
3. Cook quinoa according to package instructions.
4. Steam assorted greens and season with olive oil and lemon.

TURKEY MEATBALLS WITH TOMATO SAUCE AND ZUCCHINI NOODLES

INGREDIENTS:

- Ground turkey
- Tomato sauce or marinara
- Zucchini
- Garlic
- Herbs (such as basil and oregano)

INSTRUCTIONS:

1. Prepare turkey meatballs seasoned with garlic and herbs. Bake or pan-fry until cooked through.
2. Simmer tomato sauce with additional herbs.
3. Spiralize zucchini into noodles and lightly sauté them.
4. Serve turkey meatballs over zucchini noodles with tomato sauce.

LENTIL CURRY WITH BROWN RICE

INGREDIENTS:

- Lentils
- Brown rice
- Coconut milk
- Curry spices (turmeric, cumin, coriander)

- Onion
- Garlic
- Ginger

INSTRUCTIONS:

1. Cook lentils in coconut milk with curry spices until tender.
2. Sauté chopped onion, garlic, and ginger in a separate pan.
3. Serve lentil curry over cooked brown rice.

BAKED TOFU WITH STIR-FRIED VEGETABLES

INGREDIENTS:

- Firm tofu
- Assorted vegetables (bell peppers, broccoli, snap peas)
- Soy sauce or tamari
- Olive oil
- Herbs and spices

INSTRUCTIONS:

1. Press tofu to remove excess water, then bake until lightly golden.
2. Stir-fry assorted vegetables in olive oil and soy sauce or tamari.

3. Season tofu and vegetables with herbs and spices of your choice.

ROASTED CHICKEN WITH SWEET POTATO WEDGES AND STEAMED GREEN BEANS

INGREDIENTS:

- Chicken thighs or drumsticks
- Sweet potatoes
- Green beans
- Olive oil
- Herbs and spices

INSTRUCTIONS:

1. Rub chicken with olive oil, herbs, and spices, then roast until fully cooked.
2. Cut sweet potatoes into wedges, toss in olive oil, and roast until tender.
3. Steam green beans until crisp-tender and season to taste.

STIR-FRIED SHRIMP WITH QUINOA AND MIXED VEGETABLES

INGREDIENTS:

- Shrimp
- Quinoa
- Assorted vegetables (mushrooms, bell peppers, snap peas)
- Soy sauce or tamari
- Olive oil
- Garlic and ginger (minced)

INSTRUCTIONS:

1. Stir-fry shrimp in olive oil with minced garlic and ginger until cooked.
2. Cook quinoa according to package instructions.
3. Stir-fry assorted vegetables and season with soy sauce or tamari.
4. Serve shrimp and vegetables over cooked quinoa.

GRILLED STEAK WITH ROASTED ROOT VEGETABLES

INGREDIENTS:

- Steak cuts (such as sirloin or ribeye)
- Root vegetables (carrots, parsnips, beets)
- Olive oil
- Herbs and spices
- Balsamic glaze (optional)

INSTRUCTIONS:

1. Marinate steak with olive oil, herbs, and spices. Grill to desired doneness.
2. Toss root vegetables in olive oil, season with herbs and spices, and roast until tender.
3. Drizzle with balsamic glaze if desired before serving.

BAKED COD WITH LEMON HERB SAUCE AND QUINOA

INGREDIENTS:

- Cod fillets
- Quinoa
- Lemon
- Olive oil
- Herbs (such as parsley, dill, and thyme)

- Garlic

INSTRUCTIONS:

1. Season cod fillets with olive oil, lemon juice, minced garlic, and herbs.
2. Bake cod until it flakes easily with a fork.
3. Cook quinoa according to package instructions.
4. Prepare a lemon herb sauce with chopped herbs, lemon juice, and olive oil. Serve over baked cod and quinoa.

VEGETABLE STIR-FRY WITH BROWN RICE AND TOFU

INGREDIENTS:

- Firm tofu
- Assorted vegetables (bell peppers, broccoli, carrots)
- Brown rice
- Soy sauce or tamari
- Olive oil
- Garlic and ginger (minced)

INSTRUCTIONS:

1. Press tofu to remove excess water, then cube and stir-fry until golden.
2. Stir-fry assorted vegetables in olive oil with minced garlic and ginger.
3. Cook brown rice according to package instructions.
4. Combine tofu and vegetables, season with soy sauce or tamari, and serve over cooked brown rice.

SNACK AND SWEET RECIPES FOR GRAVES' DISEASE COOKBOOK

APPLE SLICES WITH ALMOND BUTTER

INGREDIENTS:

- Apples
- Almond butter

INSTRUCTIONS:

1. Core and slice apples into wedges.
2. Serve with a side of almond butter for dipping.

TRAIL MIX (NUTS AND DRIED FRUITS)

INGREDIENTS:

- Assorted nuts (almonds, walnuts, cashews)
- Dried fruits (raisins, cranberries, apricots)

INSTRUCTIONS:

1. Mix together assorted nuts and dried fruits in a bowl.
2. Portion into snack-sized bags for easy grab-and-go snacks.

GREEK YOGURT WITH HONEY AND WALNUTS

INGREDIENTS:

- Greek yogurt
- Honey
- Walnuts

INSTRUCTIONS:

1. Spoon Greek yogurt into a bowl.
2. Drizzle with honey and sprinkle with crushed walnuts.

RICE CAKES WITH AVOCADO SPREAD

INGREDIENTS:

- Rice cakes
- Avocado
- Lemon juice
- Salt and pepper

INSTRUCTIONS:

1. Mash avocado with lemon juice, salt, and pepper.
2. Spread over rice cakes for a healthy snack option.

COTTAGE CHEESE WITH PINEAPPLE CHUNKS

INGREDIENTS:

- Cottage cheese
- Pineapple chunks (fresh or canned)

INSTRUCTIONS:

1. Spoon cottage cheese into a bowl.
2. Top with pineapple chunks for a sweet and tangy snack.

MIXED NUTS AND DRIED FRUIT

INGREDIENTS:

- Mixed nuts (almonds, cashews, pistachios)
- Dried fruits (apricots, dates, figs)

INSTRUCTIONS:

1. Combine mixed nuts and dried fruits in a bowl.
2. Portion into snack-sized servings for a nutritious snack.

SLICED CUCUMBER WITH COTTAGE CHEESE

INGREDIENTS:

- Cucumber
- Cottage cheese

INSTRUCTIONS:

1. Slice cucumber into rounds.
2. Top each cucumber slice with a dollop of cottage cheese.

BERRIES WITH A DOLLOP OF GREEK YOGURT

INGREDIENTS:

- Mixed berries (strawberries, blueberries, raspberries)
- Greek yogurt

INSTRUCTIONS:

1. Place mixed berries in a bowl.
2. Add a dollop of Greek yogurt on top of the berries.

HANDFUL OF PUMPKIN SEEDS

INGREDIENTS:

- Pumpkin seeds (pepitas)

INSTRUCTIONS:

1. Simply grab a handful of pumpkin seeds for a quick and nutritious snack option.

APPLE SLICES WITH CINNAMON

INGREDIENTS:

- Apples
- Ground cinnamon

INSTRUCTIONS:

1. Core and slice apples into wedges.
2. Sprinkle cinnamon over the apple slices for a flavorful snack.

BEVERAGE AND SMOOTHIE RECIPES FOR GRAVES' DISEASE COOKBOOK

GREEN DETOX SMOOTHIE

INGREDIENTS:

- Spinach
- Kale
- Cucumber
- Green apple
- Lemon juice
- Ginger
- Water or coconut water

INSTRUCTIONS:

1. Blend spinach, kale, chopped cucumber, green apple, lemon juice, ginger, and water (or coconut water) until smooth.

BERRY BLAST SMOOTHIE

INGREDIENTS:

- Mixed berries (strawberries, blueberries, raspberries)
- Banana
- Greek yogurt
- Almond milk
- Honey (optional)

INSTRUCTIONS:

1. Blend mixed berries, banana, Greek yogurt, almond milk, and honey until well combined.

GOLDEN TURMERIC LATTE

INGREDIENTS:

- Turmeric powder
- Cinnamon
- Ground ginger
- Coconut milk or almond milk
- Honey (optional)

INSTRUCTIONS:

1. Heat coconut milk or almond milk in a saucepan.
2. Whisk in turmeric powder, cinnamon, ground ginger, and honey until combined. Heat but do not boil.

MINTY CUCUMBER LEMONADE

INGREDIENTS:

- Cucumber
- Fresh mint leaves
- Lemon juice
- Water
- Honey or stevia (optional)

INSTRUCTIONS:

1. Blend cucumber, fresh mint leaves, lemon juice, water, and sweetener (if desired) until smooth.
2. Strain the mixture and serve over ice.

PINEAPPLE GINGER SMOOTHIE

INGREDIENTS:

- Pineapple chunks
- Fresh ginger

- Greek yogurt or coconut yogurt
- Almond milk or coconut water

INSTRUCTIONS:

1. Blend pineapple chunks, fresh ginger, Greek yogurt (or coconut yogurt), and almond milk (or coconut water) until smooth.

CREAMY MATCHA LATTE

INGREDIENTS:

- Matcha powder
- Hot water
- Coconut milk or almond milk
- Honey or maple syrup (optional)

INSTRUCTIONS:

1. Whisk matcha powder with hot water until dissolved.
2. Heat coconut milk or almond milk separately, then combine with the matcha mixture. Sweeten if desired.

ORANGE CARROT GINGER JUICE

INGREDIENTS:

- Carrots
- Oranges
- Fresh ginger

INSTRUCTIONS:

1. Juice carrots and oranges in a juicer.
2. Blend in fresh ginger for an added kick.

PROTEIN-PACKED SPINACH SMOOTHIE

INGREDIENTS:

- Spinach
- Banana
- Protein powder (plant-based or whey)
- Almond milk or coconut water

INSTRUCTIONS:

1. Blend spinach, banana, protein powder, and almond milk (or coconut water) until smooth.

REFRESHING WATERMELON MINT COOLER

INGREDIENTS:

- Watermelon chunks
- Fresh mint leaves
- Lime juice
- Water or sparkling water

INSTRUCTIONS:

1. Blend watermelon chunks, fresh mint leaves, lime juice, and water (or sparkling water) until smooth.

BLUEBERRY LAVENDER SMOOTHIE

INGREDIENTS:

- Blueberries
- Lavender buds (culinary-grade)
- Greek yogurt or coconut yogurt
- Almond milk or coconut water

INSTRUCTIONS:

1. Blend blueberries, lavender buds, Greek yogurt (or coconut yogurt), and almond milk (or coconut water) until well combined.

CONCLUSION

This cookbook has been meticulously curated with the aim of providing individuals navigating Graves' disease with a culinary journey that not only nourishes the body but also tantalizes the taste buds. Managing Graves' disease requires a mindful approach to nutrition, and these recipes have been thoughtfully vetted and confirmed to support a balanced and health-conscious diet.

From nutrient-dense meals to delightful snacks and refreshing beverages, each recipe within these pages has been designed to offer a fusion of flavors while considering the specific dietary needs associated with Graves' disease. Incorporating a variety of wholesome ingredients, these recipes aim to not only satiate hunger but also promote wellness and vitality.

We understand the challenges that come with managing Graves' disease, and our commitment lies in providing a collection of well-vetted, confirmed, and delightful culinary options to inspire and empower individuals on their health journey. We encourage you to explore, experiment, and savor these dishes, finding joy in nourishing your body while enjoying the pleasures of the table.

May this cookbook be a companion on your path toward optimal health and well-being, celebrating the union of good food and a vibrant life.

Eat well, stay well.